Erectile Dysfunction Cure

The Ultimate Guide To Naturally And Permanently Cure Erectile Dysfunction

By Michael Cesar

Table of Contents

Introduction

I want to thank you and congratulate you for purchasing this book, *Erectile Dysfunction Cure.*

This book contains proven steps and strategies on how to naturally and permanently cure erectile dysfunction.

Throughout this book, you will learn about alternative methods to treat ED. These methods focus on the whole body, not just your ED. You are more than your ED, and your ED treatment needs to address more than your ED. Alternative ED treatments use a holistic approach that lead to a fuller quality of life.

These treatments include:

- Journaling
- The Sedona Method
- Meditation
- Acupuncture
- Tantra
- Ayurveda
- Other methods such as herbal supplements and diet modification

By using these methods, you will open yourself up to a fullness of life that was not possible in the midst of your experience with ED. While ED is a common condition, your treatment options don't have to be common. You don't have to rely upon the traditional prescription medication choices. More and more healthcare providers are suggesting complementary and alternative medicine choices for the treatment of ED.

The purpose of this book is to make you aware of such options so that you can make knowledgeable choices regarding the treatment of your ED. Treating your ED is about regaining control over your life, and this control begins with informed decision making.

Thanks again for downloading this book. I hope you enjoy it!

Chapter 1: Addressing the Elephant in the Room

Erectile dysfunction, the inability to achieve or sustain an erection, is a subject that makes men uncomfortable. For one thing, there's the need for privacy. ED involves the penis, and that's a subject that is private for most men. Another reason that ED discussions make men uncomfortable is because of embarrassment or shame. The ability to achieve and sustain an erection is, in most men's eyes, directly tied to sexual performance. Society places so much pressure on a man to be virile. From an early age, men are exposed to society's ideal of manliness by sexual prowess and that experiencing ED is taken as a sign of weakness. A man suffering from ED may feel guilty for not being able to sexually please his partner. For all of these reasons and so many more, erectile dysfunction has become the elephant in the room, but it doesn't have to be this way.

Removing the Stigma

If you are suffering from ED, you are not alone:

- At least 30 million men in America suffer from some degree of erectile dysfunction.
- It's also reported that 40% of men in their 40s reported having occasional erectile dysfunction.
- It's been estimated that 70% of men that have ED don't seek medical treatment.
- Talk with your partner.
- Talk with your doctor.
- There might be a medical reason behind your ED.

Causes of ED

ED can be caused by a physiological or a psychological issue. It's important to know and address the cause.

Physical Causes of ED:

- Obesity
- Atherosclerosis (hardened arteries due to plaque build-up)
- High blood pressure
- High cholesterol

- Heart disease
- COPD
- Low testosterone levels
- Diabetes
- Liver disease
- Spinal cord or nervous system disorders
- Pelvic injury
- Prescription or over-the-counter medicine usage

These underlying medical issues are a reason to seek medical attention. Treating the underlying medical issue should alleviate ED.

Psychological Causes:

- Depression
- Anxiety
- Stress
- Emotional disorders
- Fatigue
- Lack of desire/attraction
- Unspoken confusion regarding attraction to the opposite sex

Unlike physical causes of ED, psychological causes of ED can't be easily detected. To get to the root of psychological causes takes some deep introspection, which will be discussed in more detail later.

Other Causes of ED

In addition to physical and psychological causes, there are causes of ED that are a combination of the two. Tobacco use has been attributed as a cause for ED. The same goes for drinking alcohol or taking recreational drugs. These causes combine both psychological and physiological aspects.

Traditional Treatment Methods

In addition to treating the underlying causes, there are many methods available to assist with the actual symptom of ED. These methods can help you have an erection and participate in intercourse. Traditionally, such methods involved either drug therapy, vacuum devices, or even surgery. While these treatment options have been successful, these methods do have their drawbacks. For one thing, the cost factor is considerable. Two, you have to consider the invasiveness of these procedures. Finally, you have to consider whether or not these therapies are aligned with your philosophy of life.

Alternative Medicine Treatments

But are these the only treatment options that are available for sufferers of ED? No, they are not. Natural cures for ED exist and have several advantages. These treatments are non-invasive and are safe. They provide a variety of choices that's not offered by traditional therapies. Most importantly, natural ED treatments gives you control over your treatment options. You pick which treatment is best aligned with your philosophy of life. You take ownership of your treatment. You become a participant in your treatment, instead of having something done to you.

In essence, you're taking back ownership of your life, not just your ED. Treating your ED is more than just fixing a problem. It's about enjoying life to the fullest and being fully aware of that experience. By choosing a natural cure, you're able to do this without having to rely on medical contrivances to do it. Natural therapies give you the freedom to participate and evolve through your treatment that doesn't exist within traditional therapies.

The Elephant in the Room Isn't Even an Elephant

As you can see, ED doesn't have to be a taboo subject. It's your body, and your body is not taboo. You should feel free to talk about it. You should feel free to do something about it. Take ownership of your body. Take ownership of your treatment.

By choosing a natural method for treating ED, you enter into a holistic treatment that is about more than your ED. *You* are more than your ED. Holistic treatment goes beyond your ED to the realization of the worth of your entire being. Yes, you should speak with a doctor about your ED, but there are a growing number of doctors that are turning to complementary and alternative medicine as a better solution for healthcare issues. Find a doctor who supports holistic therapies and find a doctor that supports you and your participation in the restoration of your body to full health. Natural methods for treating ED is not a procedure, it's a journey. Begin your journey.

Chapter 2: The Power of Journaling

Life can be hectic. You have so many responsibilities and obligations. Time, money, and other resources are limited. You have a family to love and support. You have so much to do, and there's only so much time in a day to get them done.

Add to this the frustration and other negative emotions that are compounded by erectile dysfunction, and you've become a pressure cooker. Physical symptoms aren't the only effects of ED. ED can cause anxiety, depression, and a low quality of life. Keeping your feelings inside only makes the situation worse. You have to find a way to express these feelings. You need a therapeutic release. Also, with the demands of the day pressing down on you, you need to make time to reflect upon what is happening to you and why it's happening. There are benefits to this type of introspection.

Fortunately, there is a therapeutic method that addresses all of these needs with one activity. It's cheap. It's easy. It's been around for thousands of years, but it's only been in the last hundred years or so that it's come to be regarded as an effective method for dealing with emotional or psychological issues. It's writing in a journal.

Journaling and ED
Journaling about your ED will provide you with many benefits. First of all, journaling brings a sense of clarity to your thoughts and life. The simple act of recording your thoughts daily brings a sense of order to your thoughts. With so much going on in your head, journaling allows you to focus on your ED.

Journaling and Expression
Not only does journaling bring clarity, but journaling gives you an opportunity to express your feelings regarding ED. If you're finding that you yet to have the confidence to talk to someone else about your experience, you can write it down. It's your journal, so it's going to be confidential. Or

you can choose to share it with your partner. Allowing your partner to read your journal can be a way of overcoming the desire to hide your feelings about ED. This can be a great way to open up communication with your partner. Let your partner read your journal, and then discuss what you've been feeling.

Journaling and Realization

If you are suffering from ED, you need an outlet that allows you to express your emotions instead of keeping them tucked away inside you. Expressing your feelings will help in addressing these feelings. The first step in dealing with negative emotions is admitting that they exist. Journaling can help you express these feelings. You may not even realize how you feel about ED until you write it down.

Journaling and Acceptance

Once you've written in your journal, read back through it. You'll be surprised to discover that this is your reality. Journaling helps you accept your situation. It promotes understanding and growth. Writing about your ED helps you develop a sense of self-awareness that you didn't have before you started journaling. That being said, the only cost to journaling, apart from pen and paper, is time and effort. If you're going to keep a journal about your

ED, you'll have to determine within yourself to write daily and honestly.

Journaling as a Record

In addition to journaling being a source of emotional release, journaling provides a record of your experience with ED. This information is valuable to discovering the source of your ED. Sharing this information with your healthcare provider will make the process of identifying the cause of ED simpler because as your journal patterns develop, you will include certain types of information. Your healthcare provider is going to want to know your medical history and details about your lifestyle to help make informed suggestions as to possible treatment methods. Having this information recorded in your journal will allow this information to be readily available for your healthcare provider. It provides a more detailed picture of your current situation and how you arrived to be in this situation.

What to Write About

There are many different things that you should include in your journal. Of course, one of the bits of information that you need to include in your journal is when you experience ED. You need to be specific. Include when and where it happened.

Also, include what your day was like prior to the occurrence.

Physical Description

Describe your physical condition. Were you feeling fatigued? Were you experiencing any other physical issues before the occurrence? How were you feeling physically? Keeping a record of any issues you were experiencing before and at the time of your experience with ED will aid in establishing a pattern of your physiological condition. For example, if you include the fact that you had a headache or felt dizzy, you can point to an underlying physical cause of your ED.

Mental Description

In addition to any physical issues you experience, you'll also want to include any mental or emotional issues in your journal. Were you feeling stressed? Were you anxious about something? Have you been depressed? Have you recently experienced an emotional event such as the loss of a loved one? Detailing this aspect of your life can help you and your healthcare provider determine any psychological/emotional causes of ED.

Being Honest

The key to successful journaling about your ED is to be honest. The more honesty you put on the page, the more accurate a depiction of your experience will be recorded. With this honest description, you'll be able to discover what triggered your ED. You can also discover how you actually feel about your ED. You may even discover any sexual issues you may have.

Journaling is About Discovery

The point of journaling is not to point fingers, but to discover what is causing your ED and how your ED is affecting you. You may be thinking that you know yourself pretty well, but sometimes we do such a good job at hiding our true selves from others that we even hide it from ourselves. We project an image of ourselves that we want others to see, and somehow we get ourselves caught up in that image. Or we just outright deny our true feelings. Either way, sometimes you have to force yourself into taking a realistic look in the mirror. Journaling is a means of doing that.

Journaling is an Honest Representation, Not a Bad One

Even though journaling provides you with an honest representation of your current state, it doesn't have to be negative. How you react to what you discover is totally up to you. Any healing that is possible for you has to begin with accepting your situation. Then, you have to let go of any feelings of guilt or shame. These emotions will only hinder your healing. Negative emotions weaken the immune system and cause your body to malfunction.

Whatever the cause of your ED, you have to let go of any negative emotions and free yourself to be able to move forward. If your ED was caused by destructive habits, such as smoking or drinking, determine within yourself to put an end to these habits.

Addressing the Cause of ED

Addressing the cause of your ED will cure your ED. Journaling is a powerful tool that can help you:

- Identify the causes of your ED
- Express the emotions you're feeling because of your ED
- Vent your frustrations with your ED
- Relieve any stress that ED is causing you
- Describe your experiences with ED, so that your healthcare provider gets an accurate description of your situation
- Accept the causes of your ED
- Quit any destructive habits that could possibly cause your ED.

With so many positive benefits gained from journaling, today is a good day to start journaling. Simply begin with the moment your ED began and work your way forward. Add to your journal each day. Add to your journal as new thoughts about your ED come to you. An old Chinese saying says that, "The journey of a thousand miles begins with a single step." Take that step and start journaling your way into understanding ED and your response to it.

Chapter 3: Finding Psychological Release—The Sedona Method

Your psychological makeup holds powerful sway over your physical body. It's already been noted that there are several different psychological/emotional causes of ED. To free yourself from these psychological/emotional causes, you have to find a way to release yourself from negative emotions so that they are not negatively impacting your body. In other words, if the cause of your ED is psychological/emotional, you won't be cured of your ED until you find a way to eliminate the control that this cause has on your body. To cure the cause is to cure the ED.

To cure the psychological cause of ED, you have to find a means of releasing yourself out of the psychological entanglement that you find yourself in, whether it's depression, anxiety, stress, or some other emotional issue. Sure, there are medications for dealing with psychological/emotional issues, but then you're dependent upon the medication to find that release. Instead, there's an alternative that can help you loosen the control that negative feelings can have on your body. It's called the Sedona Method.

What is the Sedona Method?

The Sedona Method is a simple, easy-to-learn technique that helps you let go of negative, unwanted feelings that you are currently feeling so that you can move past them into a productive life. The Sedona Method was first used by Lester Levinson, who was only given three months to live. Levinson created a way to release himself from the control of hurtful emotions, and in doing so, he found himself living another 42 years! Levinson's student, Hal Dwoskin, then wrote *The Sedona Method* as a how-to guide to walk others through the healing path that Levinson took.

The key to the Sedona Method is letting go of the unwanted feeling. Also, the Sedona Method needs to be applied in the immediate context of feeling that negative emotion. Once you realize that you're experiencing a negative feeling, that's when it's time to apply the Sedona Method.

The Sedona Method is nothing more than a series of questions that guides you through working out your feelings. The problem with negative feelings is that we often don't let them go. We may tell ourselves that we've let them go, but they remain hidden in our unconscious waiting to return at an inopportune time. The longer these emotions stay pushed down, the worse the situation will be when they are finally expressed. By dealing with the emotion in the moment, you keep the situation from worsening. The outcome is that you're free to move past the emotion and return to an enjoyable level of life.

Interestingly, negative emotions are usually the result of an unfulfilled, unspoken desire like approval, control, or safety. Addressing the emotion allows you to confront the desire. Ultimately, by confronting the desire by reflecting upon the felt emotion, you are actually able to fulfill the desire in a healthy manner.

Sometimes, we feel as if our emotions are controlling us. The only reason this is true is because we've allowed this situation to be. These emotions are yours, and you are in control of them. By working through these emotions, you will gain acceptance, control, safety, or whatever desire that you feel is unfulfilled. It'll just be in a manner that is different than what you thought you needed to fulfill that desire. The Sedona Method allows you to process all of your emotions and desires and master them so that you can move past them.

The Sedona Method Process

To begin the Sedona Method, focus on your situation. Open yourself up to the negative emotions. Be honest with yourself. Hiding these feelings won't make them go away. Neither will rationalizing them. Feel them in the moment. You have to become in tune with your inner self. Knowing how you feel and why is important to the process. Think about your state of being before you began to feel this way. This sets up a division of what your life is like without the issue, and what it's like with the issue.

If you're dealing with an issue from the past, think back to that time. Remember how you felt. Rely upon the pictures that are conjured up in your mind as it drifts back to that time. Allow yourself to feel those feelings again in the current moment. Think about what your life was like before this issue. Be with the feeling, welcome the feeling, and stay with the feeling.

Next, ask yourself a series of questions. The purpose of the questions isn't even to arrive at an answer. The purpose of the questions is to get you thinking through your emotions. They are simple yes or no type questions that prepare you for letting go of the painful emotion. It's the final step that is important.

It's important to welcome the feelings that arise. Welcome that feeling into the moment and allow it to be. Embrace the feeling before going into the questions. Remember that the questions can be answered by a yes or no answer, and that the answer isn't really the focus. The answer is just a means of getting to a place of release. Continue through the process until the end. If you don't yet feel that release, repeat the process as many times as you need until you find that release.

The questions are:
1. Could I let this feeling go? Could I allow this feeling to be here? Could I welcome this feeling?
2. Am I willing to let this feeling go?
3. When?

If you answer yes to the first two questions and your answer to the third question is now, you're ready to release that feeling. Take a deep breath. As you exhale, release that feeling out of your body and feel the release. If you're answer was no or not yet, continue with the method until you can answer yes. Then, release the feeling as you exhale.

It's the final question that you need to focus on. The other two just prepare you. Asking yourself when puts you in the immediate present with that emotion. It works like a sort of invitation to release yourself from that emotion. It suggests to you that you don't have to be controlled by this feeling forever. Freedom from this negative emotion is possible and is available to you.

If you don't find yourself feeling released, keep asking yourself when. Keep the thought of breakthrough a constant in your thoughts. As you repeat that last question, you begin to sense a gradual release. This is okay. You probably have layers of this emotion that have developed without you realizing. You have to work through each layer.

The good news is that once you've released yourself from the emotion, it doesn't come back. A new instance of it might, but that old experience is done with, and you've moved on. If a new instance arises, deal with it the same way as you did previously. Work your way through the Sedona Method until you've felt a release.

The Sedona Method and ED

Now, you may be asking yourself, "What does the Sedona Method have to do with ED?" The answer is that the Sedona Method is an effective way in addressing the psychological/emotional causes of ED.

Take anxiety for instance. If you're feeling anxious about something, then your chance of experiencing ED is elevated. If you want to minimize this chance, you can use the Sedona Method to release you from that anxious feeling. The moment you begin to feel anxious about something, work your way through the Sedona Method. Overtime, you will begin to see that your overall anxiety level has been reduced. The same will be true for other negative emotions you may be feeling that may be causing your ED. It's also true for any negative attitudes, unfulfilled desires, or obsessive fantasies. The Sedona Method works on any negative aspect of your thought life. You can even use it as a means of releasing yourself from excessive pornographic addiction, if you need to gain control over that aspect of your life.

You can use the Sedona Method to release yourself from negative past experiences. Bring that experience into the present by thinking back to the moment of that experience. Let the scene play in your head. Then, work your way through the Sedona Method. Repeat the method until you feel released from that prior negative experience. Letting go of something in the past will allow you to be free in the present. This will help you with any past negative experiences that might be causing your ED.

Finally, you can use the Sedona Method to move past any negative feelings that are being caused by ED like a sense of guilt or frustration. When you feel these emotions, apply the Sedona Method. You don't have to feel bad about experiencing ED. It is a natural occurrence that happens to a large percentage of the male population. Using the Sedona Method can free you from feeling any negative emotions you might have about suffering from ED.

The Sedona Method Helps You Live in the Moment

By being in constant contact with your inner self, you can be free to live in the moment. It shifts the focus off of your psychological/emotional state and onto your current situation. This can be freeing during moments of intimacy. You're no longer focused on what has been bothering you. You're now free to enjoy your current experience because you've distanced yourself from your problems for good. They no longer control you. You control your emotions. You are now released to enjoy your life in all of its many wondrous aspects.

Chapter 4: Meditation: A Prepared Mind Against ED

As the world grows more technologically advanced, it seems that the pressures of the day are increasing instead of decreasing. Instead of freeing up our time for enjoyment, we seem to cram more responsibilities into the time that has been freed up by technology. Technology has increased productivity, and increased productivity has required more from us.

Effects of Negative Emotions on the Brain
This increased productivity puts a strain on your mental faculties. Your brain is like a muscle. When you over-exert a muscle, you strain it, and it doesn't function properly. When you over exert the

brain, it loses control over the functions of your body.

Stress, anxiety, and frustration worsen the situation. You lose the ability to cope, to function, and to perform. This loss of ability affects your sexual drive. It's all connected because it's all centered in the brain. It's also connected because it's all centered in your life energy. If the stresses of the day zap your life energy, it's going to affect all aspects of your life, including your sexual drive.

Think About It, Seriously

So what can be done to combat this wear and tear on your mental faculties and on your life energy? First of all, you need to heal the damage already done. Secondly, you need to strengthen your brain and life energy so that it can withstand the pressures of this life. Going back to the muscle analogy, when you've strained a muscle, it needs to heal. You put PRICE into practice: protection, rest, ice, compression, and elevation. Once the muscle strain has healed, you take preventive measures to properly strengthen the muscle so that strain doesn't happen again.

The same goes for when your brain and energy is overworked. You take steps to heal and prevent. Fortunately, for your brain and life energy, the healing and strengthening can be accomplished with the same method: meditation.

The Positive Effects of Meditation

Meditation is not a new gimmick. People have been practicing meditation for thousands of years, yet it's only been recently that meditation has become an accepted form of healing. With an ever-growing turn to complementary and alternative medicine, more and more research has been conducted into the positive effects of meditation for health and wellness. And this research has shown that meditation does work to provide healing and stimulate positive health gains in several different ways.

First of all, meditation helps reduce stress and anxiety. Meditation allows you to take your focus off outside stimulus and focus it within. This focus allows your life energy to be focused on your body instead of it being focused on outside pressures. This frees up the mind to begin to direct the body to work on itself.

Thus, your body can:
- Reduce tension
- Gain focus
- Improve metabolism
- Strengthen your immune system
- Improve your sleep cycles

- Lower blood pressure
- Improve oxygen levels in the blood
- Increase energy levels.

In effect, meditation heals the mind so that the mind can heal the body.

Not only does meditation heal the body, but meditation also strengthens your willpower. According to Kelly McGonigal, a professor at Stanford, your willpower stems from your pre-frontal cortex. Research into meditation reveals that individuals who practice meditation show an increase in gray matter in the pre-frontal cortex and increased neural connections. In other words, meditation strengthens your brain. This is the preventative side of meditation.

Finally, meditation helps you focus your life energy. With your energy pulled in many different directions, you begin to feel the strain of the imbalance. With drained energy, you feel disconnected from others, from the world, and from yourself. Realigning your energy will bring you back into connection. You can then turn that energy toward your sex drive. Sexual energy is derived from your overall life energy. If your life energy is out of balance, your sexual energy will also be out of balance.

Meditation and ED

Since meditation is a means of healing your body, a sort of training for your brain, and a method for focusing your sexual energy, it makes sense that meditation can help you cure your ED. For one thing, the slowed heart rate and lowered blood pressure will provide better blood flow, which is necessary for engorgement. The increased focus and self-awareness will boost the ability of your male organs to function properly. Training your mind through meditation allows you to stay focused during sexual encounters by removing distractions.

All of these benefits of meditation for treating ED have been researched. One study sampled 9 men who were experiencing ED. During the pre-study interview, all of the men mentioned that prior to experiencing ED, they felt a feeling of warmth in their genitals when they were beginning to become aroused. They also mentioned noticing a lack of this warm feeling since experiencing ED.

During the study, the men were trained by a doctor on how to meditate by focusing on their breathing. Once in a meditative state, the men were instructed to concentrate on their male organs and imagine that feeling of warmth returning to their genitals. The men were then sent home with instructions to practice this meditation twice a day for 15 minutes. Within two weeks' time, the majority of the men were able to function normally during sex. Only two men didn't achieve satisfactory results because they weren't even able to achieve a meditative state due to lack of focus. After 3 months, the men returned back and reported continued normal sexual functioning.

Tips and Techniques

You can achieve the same results as the men who participated in the study. It's a matter of being motivated enough to set aside two 15-minute periods daily for meditation. During this time of meditation, you'll focus all of your energy on your sexual desire and genitals. Be sure to keep your thoughts pure. Unwholesome thoughts distract. Below are some techniques that you can use to meditate and overcome your ED.

Achieving a Meditative State:

1. Rhythmic Breathing

   a. Get in a comfortable position somewhere free from distractions.
   b. Get still and stay still. Put distance between you and your urge to move.
   c. Focus on your breathing. Either close your eyes or pick a spot in front of you to focus on. Bring attention to

your breathing. As you breathe in say, "Inhale" out loud. As you breathe out, say, "Exhale" out loud. You can eventually move to saying this within yourself. Do this until you can focus on your breathing without saying the words. Then, just pay attention to the air going in and out of your nose/mouth.

d. Keep your focus on your breathing. Fight the urge to fall asleep.

2. Deep Breathing. This is also called belly breathing.

   a. Imagine a spot just below your belly button.
   b. Imagine air filling that spot.
   c. Let air fill that spot while focusing on your abdomen expanding.
   d. Release the air like you would let air out of a balloon.
   e. Repeat this until your focus is inward.

3. Progressive Relaxation

   a. Focus on breathing.
   b. Close your eyes.
   c. Mentally scan your body.
   d. Notice any areas that feel tense or cramped.
   e. Loosen these areas.
   f. Let go of as much tension as you can.

g. Focus on a pleasant thought.

4. Mental Imagery Relaxation. This is sort of like a mental escape.

   a. Relax.
   b. Focus on your breathing.
   c. Think of a pleasant sexual experience with your partner. Remember to keep it wholesome.
   d. Focus on the experience: the feelings, the touches, and the outcome.
   e. Play it back in your mind.
   f. Allow your energy to be turned inward.

5. Positive Affirmations

   a. Focus on your breathing.
   b. Repeat positive affirmations to yourself.
   c. You can say things like, "I'm letting go of the things I can't control." Or, "All my needs are met." Or, "I can handle anything that comes my way."
   d. As you repeat this affirmation, focus your attention and energy inward.
   e. Believe what you are saying.

Once You've Achieved a Meditative State

Once you're in a meditative state, begin to focus on your sexual organs. Imagine a feeling of warmth beginning to radiate. Imagine your organs functioning properly. Imagine you and your partner successfully consummating.

Focus your attention and energy on arousal. It's not about ejaculation. It's about the fulfillment you realize through orgasm. It's about enjoying the entire experience. Keep your focus inward on the pleasure that sex brings. Don't allow yourself to be distracted. If you do this twice daily for 15 minutes each, you will begin to experience results. You'll also find that the joy of sex has returned.

You'll also receive all of the physical benefits of meditation. Meditation works, if you can control your mind through focus. The self-awareness that you gain from meditation is powerful, if you can channel your energy inward.

Chapter 5: Tantra and ED

Up until this point, we have discussed ways of taking on your ED through the mind. While these may work for some, others may need to go further and include the body. This is especially true if you have a physical cause to your ED. You need to bring your mind and your body into alignment.

Often times, your mind becomes disconnected from your body. Distractions arise daily within your life that takes your focus off your body and places it on something else. With your mind and body disconnected, you are no longer in control of what is happening within your body. This is true for ED. You are no longer in control of your body's reaction to sexual stimulus. You have to realign your body and mind to be able to control your body and enjoy sexual pleasure again. This requires a method that focuses both on the body and the mind, and this is what tantra does.

Tantra: Aligning the Body and the Mind

Aligning the body, mind, and spirit has been practiced for over 5,000 years. During this time, practitioners of tantra have learned how to channel their energy into their sexuality, thus opening themselves up to a heightened level of awareness and increased sensory perception of the experience.

The word tantra is from Sanskrit and literally means "to weave together." Yes, sometimes it is applied using a sexual metaphor as in the joining of partners, but this is only meant as a representation. More to the point, tantra is the weaving together of the mind, body, and spirit. It's the alignment of all of your various aspects to channel your energy in the right direction.

Tantra provides a vehicle of self-awareness by increasing your focus inward. By increasing your focus inward, you are able to harness your energy to make things happen in your body. Ultimately, tantra is about regaining control over your body. It's your body, and what you experience in your body is under your control. With tantra, you become the source of your own pleasure. Even in the midst of an intimate encounter with your partner, you are still the master of your own ecstasy. You're sexual ecstasy comes from within, and with tantra you tap into that inner self to channel your energy into your sexual experience.

Thus, tantra is about experiencing sexuality fully. It's not about the end result. It's about the process by which you arrive at the end result. Yes, tantra does make use of the orgasm, but most tantric teaching is about achieving orgasm without ejaculation. It's about preserving and strengthening your sexual energy, not about depleting it. In doing this, it takes the whole person into account. The focus of unifying the body, mind, and spirit makes tantra an excellent method for addressing your ED, since ED affects the whole person.

How Tantra Helps with ED

Within tantric teachings, you learn that you are the creator of your experience. In the case of ED, you can be the source of your freedom from ED. Tantric teaching also asserts the value of living in the moment. In regards to ED, this is the moment of a sexual encounter. Tantra allows you to focus on the moment while eliminating any distractions or blocks that stand in the way of your fulfillment.

Tantra trains you to fully embrace the sensuality of the moment and focus your energy into that moment. In so doing, you focus on what your body is experiencing in the moment and are aware of sensory perception. Your mind is connected with your body and your life energy. You then take this alignment and channel it into your sexual energy. By focusing on the process of channeling your energy, you remove inhibitions, mental blocks, and negative emotions that have arisen in your being and stand in the way of you enjoying the moment.

The Basics of Tantra

Part of the awareness that you gain through tantra is the awareness of your body's energy system, the chakra system. There are 7 energy centers in the body: the area near your genitals, the lower belly, below the diaphragm, the heart, the throat, around the eyebrows, and near the top of your head.

The 3 keys to accessing your chakras are breathing, sound vibrations, and movement. By combining these 3 keys, your focus will be turned inward and then you can channel your energy toward your sexuality. Interestingly, tantra takes the concept behind the meditation technique discussed in the previous practice and goes one step further by adding the movement.

In dealing with ED, you need to open two chakras: the root chakra and the sacral chakra. The root chakra is located at the base of your spine, which is your coccyx. It's accessed through the perineum, the area between your anus and your scrotum. The root chakra is associated with the feelings of safety and being grounded. This energy is important for treating ED because it helps you ground yourself and allows for growth as a person. The sacral chakra is located around the pelvic bone just above your sexual organs. This energy is the center of your sexuality, and is vital to overcoming ED.

Tantric Methods to Help Overcome ED

Breathing Techniques

Breathing and arousal go hand in hand because they are both controlled by the parasympathetic nervous system. The parasympathetic nervous system works to slow down breathing and to lower the heart rate. It also causes erections. By activating the parasympathetic nervous system with controlled breathing in a relaxed state, you can achieve erectile function. So, with that being said, here are some tantric breathing techniques.

1) Deep Belly Breathing

   a) Breathe deeply and slowly from the diaphragm while in a relaxed state.
   b) Inhale through the nose and exhale through the mouth.
   c) As you exhale through the mouth, let out a sound that feels good to you. It may be a sigh. This will help you focus on your breathing and the energy you are channeling. Continue to breathe like this until you are in a relaxed state.

2) Sipping Breath (It's kind of like sipping through a straw without the straw.)

   a) Sip in breaths through pursed lips as you inhale.
   b) Imagine you are drawing energy up through the center of your body, up from the perineum to the crown of your head.
   c) As you exhale, imagine the energy going back down to your perineum.

3) Long Deep Breath

   a) In a relaxed state, sitting cross-legged, take a deep belly breath and hold it there, by arching your back and pushing your chest out. You can place the palm of your hands onto your knees to support you.
   b) Hold the breath briefly.

c) Let the breath out by contracting your diaphragm all the way and straightening the back.
d) Repeat the process for several breaths.

4) Breath of Fire

a) Start with the Long Breath
b) When you go to exhale, as the air is going out, immediately inhale and fill the abdomen back up with air.
c) Continue doing this and establish a rhythm.

Muscle Strengthening Movements

While helping to focus your energy in your root chakra, these exercises will also strengthen muscles in this area.

1) PC Muscle Exercise: Your pubococcygeus muscles are the muscles that make up your pelvic floor. These are the muscles used to stop urination.

a) Imagine that you're trying to stop urination. Flex your PC muscles and hold them for 5 seconds.
b) Repeat about 10−15 times.
c) Do this twice a day.
d) If you're contracting your PC muscles properly, you should feel your testicles rise.

2) Pelvic Rocking: Awaken the energy in your root and sacral chakras.

    a) Lie down on a firm surface.
    b) Bend your knees with your feet placed on the floor, hip-width apart.
    c) Inhale, and as you do, rock your tailbone down while arching your back
    d) Your buttocks will rise slightly off the floor.
    e) Exhale and lower to starting position.
    f) Focus on the root chakra while doing this.

3) Testicular Elevations

    a) Sit on the edge of a chair or stand with your feet shoulder-width apart.
    b) Raise and lower your testicles.
    c) At first, you may need to use abdominal muscles, but eventually you'll be able to do this using only the pelvic muscles.
    d) Inhale as you raise them. Exhale as you lower them.
    e) Focus on the energy in the root chakra.

4) Practice Sexual Continence

    a) A key thought with tantra is that ejaculation expels sexual energy.
    b) By holding back ejaculation, you increase your libido.
    c) Let your focus be on the total experience during sex and not just on finishing.

d) Relax your mind and focus on the energy that is being channeled to your genitals.
e) Enjoy the experience and hold out as long as you can.

Massage Techniques

There are several methods of massage that will help you overcome ED. The point of the massage is to stimulate your sexual organs to be receptive to sexual energy. The purpose of these massages is not orgasm. It's a preparatory step to achieving a fuller orgasm. A key to the success of the massage is relaxation. Focus on the energy being channeled. Practice your breathing. You can perform these massages on yourself, or you can have your partner perform them on you. Be sure to use massage oil that is natural and that is pleasing to you. Some commonly used massage oils are coconut, sunflower, or sweet almond oil. Relax and allow yourself to feel the pleasure. It's good for you.

Lingam Massage

1) Lie down naked on a flat surface in a location free of distractions and conducive to relaxation.
2) Enter a relaxed state (Use rhythmic breathing, meditation, or whatever method used to achieve relaxation).
3) You may want to prepare for the lingam massage by massaging the tops of your legs and

your navel area. This helps you get into the moment of the lingam massage.

4) While practicing your breathing exercises, massage your lingam. Vary the patterns of the strokes and the pressure.
   a) Be sure to massage the entire lingam. Massage the base, the shaft, the top, and the testicles.
   b) You can massage the lingam with one hand while massaging the testicles with the other.
5) Focus on the energy you are experiencing in your lingam.
6) Pay attention to what is happening to it as you massage.
7) Note every sense you experience. Listen to your breaths. Concentrate on what your skin is feeling. Add sounds to your breathing. The more senses you involve, the more in tune you'll be with the experience.
8) Imagine the sexual energy that you feel in your lingam spreading through your spine upward and all over your body.
9) Continue this until aroused.

External Prostate Massage through the Perineum

1) Lie naked on a firm surface with your knees up and feet down flat.
2) Practice breathing exercises and put yourself in a relaxed state.
3) Find the spot on your perineum between your scrotum and anus.
4) Adding a little pressure, massage this area using circular motions.

5) While doing so, focus on your breathing and channeling your energy to your root and sacral chakras.

<u>Internal Prostate Massage</u>

While the external prostate massage may work for some, others may have to rely on the internal prostate massage, which is done through the anus. It may be uncomfortable to some at first. This is why proper breathing and relaxation are important. Internal prostate exam allows for better access to the prostate than the external massage.

1) Lie naked on a firm surface with your knees bent and extended outward slightly with feet flat about hip-width apart.
2) Begin with breathing and relaxation methods.
3) Perform lingam massage to achieve further relaxation.
4) Lubricate the anus in a manner that is pleasurable such as a circular motion.
5) Apply gentle and firm pressure to the anus with a fingertip.
6) Once the finger has been received into the anus, give the muscles time to adjust.
7) Find the prostate, a round protrusion about 2 inches from the rectum.
8) Massage the prostate with various motions until erection is achieved.

Aligning the Body, Mind, and Spirit

Tantra is about whole body alignment. It does cause heightened sexual arousal. This can help you overcome ED, but to do so you need to remain relaxed and focused on your breathing. Enter fully into the experience. Disregard distractions and remove any blocks. If you keep practicing these techniques, you will find that your situation improves greatly over time. Eventually, you may continue to use these techniques, not because you need them, but because you enjoy them.

Chapter 6: Acupuncture and the Flow of Qi

Much of this book has emphasized the importance of energy, especially sexual energy in regards to ED. There's a simple reason for this. Energy is everywhere. It's in the sun that provides you light and warmth. It's in lightning that produces ozone-generating chemicals that sustain your atmosphere. It's in the fire that burns to heat your food. Getting a little more technical, it is energy that powers your computers, cellphones, or any other electrically-powered device that you use in your daily life. Energy is everywhere. It is even found within your body.

The Ancients and Energy

The ancients understood this principle. They understood that your body is sustained by a life-energy force. They also understood that a disruption in this life force would manifest in symptoms of decline or illness that would appear in your body. To alleviate these symptoms, the ancients relied on methods of restoring the flow of the life force. A blockage in the life force could be physical, psychological, or spiritual. In many regards, modern medicine is similar to ancient healing practices in that modern medicine looks for a cause of your symptoms and then a plan is created to remove that cause. Furthermore, modern medicine focuses on the same life energy as ancient healing practices.

Modern Medicine Learning from the Ancients

Consider modern medicine for a moment. So much research has been conducted on the cardiovascular and nervous systems. For modern medicine, these two systems represent the core of life because these two systems cause your body to function. In essence, they are your life force. Modern medicine simply doesn't use that terminology. Modern medicine took a page from the ancients and is trying to provide a scientific explanation for something the ancients knew about for thousands of years. There's an old saying, "The life is in the blood," and it's true. With the current push to reduce reliance upon synthetic drugs, many modern healthcare practitioners are beginning to look back to these ancient practices of healing as a method for health improvement. Acupuncture is one such ancient treatment that is receiving quite a bit of attention today in regards to alternative medical treatment, especially for ED.

Acupuncture and the Life Force

Acupuncture is a staple of Traditional Chinese Medicine. In TCM, it is believed that your life force, or *qi*, flows throughout the body along 14 invisible channels called meridians. A blockage in this flow will cause symptoms to occur. Different areas along these meridians respond to different parts of the body. To relieve symptoms, acupuncture uses the insertion of threadlike needles to the area along the affected meridian that corresponds to the part of the body in which symptoms are manifesting. The goal of the treatment is for this blockage to be removed and for energy to flow back properly to the affected areas, thus removing the symptom.

The Effects of Acupuncture Treatment

- Restores balance between sympathetic and parasympathetic nervous systems
- Stimulates nerves, muscles, and connective tissue
- Increases blood flow
- Induces relaxation response
- Releases endorphins and neurotransmitters
- Increases libido
- Eases stress, tension, anxiety, frustration, and fear

Acupuncture and ED

Because of these benefits, acupuncture can be an effective treatment for ED. As discussed in earlier chapters, increased blood flow and balance in the nervous system are needed for effective relief from ED. The endorphins and neurotransmitters helps by increasing positive feelings. Relaxation is vital to reducing the effects of stress and other negative emotions. It also aids in an increased focus.

The effectiveness of the ability of acupuncture to treat ED has been the subject of numerous studies. The overall consensus of these studies is that acupuncture cures ED in around 70% of all cases. Because of these findings, acupuncture has gained prominence in the healthcare arena as a viable alternative treatment for ED.

What to Expect from Acupuncture ED Treatment

To treat ED, a qualified acupuncture practitioner will first perform a health assessment. This involves asking you questions about your overall current state of health. These questions are geared to determine the underlying cause of your ED. In TCM terms, the practitioner is trying to determine the location of the blockage along the meridians. ED can be caused from a blockage in several different locations. In addition to questions, the practitioner will also check your pulse at the wrist, and examine your tongue. You may take comfort at knowing that during the assessment and the actual treatment sessions, you never remove your clothing. Nor does the practitioner need to examine your genitals. For acupuncture, the focus is elsewhere in the body.

Acupuncture Sessions for ED

Once the practitioner has determined the location of the energy blockage, he or she will prescribe a round of treatments. Usually, 10–20 once weekly sessions are suggested. Most ED acupuncture treatments involve inserting needles into the back, the abdomen, or your extremities. Two common places along the leg for blockages that result in impotence are the back of the knee and near the ankle. A session usually lasts around an hour.

During the Session

The session process is fairly simple. You may have to roll up your pants leg or your shirt sleeve. If the treatment involves the abdomen or back, you may have to lift up your shirt to expose that area. You then lay down comfortably on a table. Music is generally playing to help you relax. The practitioner then inserts about 5–20 needles in the prescribed area. For the next 30–40 minutes, you simply lie there and relax. Falling asleep does occur with some patients, but not always. During this time, the practitioner may manipulate the needles to stimulate the nerves. This manipulation may involve tugging on or spinning the needles. After the end of the treatment time, the acupuncturist removes the needles.

After the Session

When the needles are first inserted, you might experience a little pain that quickly subsides. Also, after the needles are removed, you might experience soreness, redness at the insertion site, or drops of blood. This is normal. You may also experience an increase of energy and a feeling of euphoria.

The risks of acupuncture are minimal. If you see a licensed acupuncturist, the needles are typically disposable, and the treatment room is sterile. Serious side effects have not been generally identified with acupuncture treatment.

Additions to Acupuncture Treatment
Along with the actual acupuncture sessions, the acupuncturist will also probably discuss food and diet with you. Acupuncture revolves around both healing diseases and maintaining positive health, but the focus is more on maintaining positive health. The practitioner may also discuss with you Qigong exercises and self-massage techniques that you can do at home to maintain the health you have obtained during your sessions. He or she may also discuss herbal supplements that you can take to aid in relieving your ED.

A Restored Life Force
The end result of acupuncture treatment for ED is a restored *qi*. Restoring the flow of your life force invigorates your sexual energy, stimulates the parasympathetic nervous system, increases blood flow, and relaxes your entire body. Free from stress and anxiety, you should be able to focus on enjoying your time with your partner. If you work to maintain this balance within your body that you have achieved through acupuncture, you will

experience a release from ED, and you will return to functioning normally. Acupuncture is an ancient method that can bring positive results to a modern condition in a safe and life-honoring manner.

Chapter 7: Ayurveda and Balancing Energies

Ayurveda is another ancient practice that has implications for use in dealing with ED. Ayurveda is a 5,000-year-old Indian healing art that focuses on holistic treatment. Many believe that Ayurveda is the oldest-known healing art. The practice of Ayurveda is still strong today, and attention toward Ayurveda is ever growing. Recent focus has shifted to Ayurveda as an alternative treatment option for ED because of its focus on the whole being, instead of just focusing on your ED.

Principles of Ayurveda

The word *Ayurveda* is from Sanskrit and means "life knowledge." According to Ayurveda practitioners, humans are a part of nature, and thus are filled with the natural elements. These elements combine to form the three basic life energies or doshas: Vata, Pitta, and Kapha. Vata is the combination of space and air. It controls blood flow and breathing and induces vitality. Pitta primarily consists of fire. It controls the metabolic processes and induces contentment. Finally, Kapha combines earth and water. It controls growth within the body, maintains the immune system, and induces love and forgiveness.

Health in your body, mind, and spirit are a balance of all three life energies. Usually, one is more dominant than the others, but a severe imbalance results in symptoms particular to which dosha, which creates our specific mental and physical characteristics, is imbalanced. Ayurveda treatment focuses on bringing balance between the doshas. There are many different types of treatment that are used by Ayurveda practitioners. A few of these are of use for treating ED.

Ayurveda Treatments for ED:

- Breathing exercises
- Massages using herbal oils
- Meditation
- Herbal medicines
- Vajikarana or aphrodisiacs

Ayurveda Discussion of ED

Interestingly, ED is a common topic among Ayurvedic texts. According to these texts, ED is an issue of vitality, thus an imbalance in the Vata Dosha. Furthermore, these texts describe how this imbalance and loss of vitality can be manifested physically, psychologically, or sexually. As for sexuality, Ayurveda holds that the body is made of seven elements, and one of these is Shukra Dhatu. It's basically a sexual reproductive tissue. For men, it's semen. According to Ayurveda, semen holds all of the essence of the three doshas. Thus, as in ancient thought, semen is the seed that bears the elements of the universe. It is present in the entire body due to its fundamental nature. An imbalance in the Shukra Dhatu will cause impotence.

How is Ayurveda Prescribed?

To begin an ayurvedic treatment for your ED, you will make a visit to an ayurvedic practitioner. During this first visit, the practitioner will check your weight, check your pulse, listen to your speech, and examine your skin, teeth, tongue, and eyes. He or she will also ask you questions pertaining to your current state of health, medical history, how your immune system is working, what you eat, how your bowels and urinary tract are working, and particulars about your lifestyle. All of this information is used to determine where the imbalance of your doshas lies. Based on this information, the practitioner will prescribe treatment methods that are specific to your situation. A tenet of Ayurveda holds that each person has a unique life signature, so causes and treatment methods will be centered on your life signature, or pulse.

Ayurvedic ED Treatment Method Specifics

Since Ayurveda has much to say about ED, there are specific treatment methods for ED for the practitioner to choose from. When discussing treatment options with your ayurvedic practitioner, speak honestly with him or her. Express your opinions regarding these treatment options. Ask questions and gain as much information as possible. Play an active role in your treatment.

Once an ayurvedic provider has assessed your current state, he or she will then detail a treatment plan that is geared specifically to you. Once again, Ayurveda takes into consideration your unique situation to determine the best treatment path for you. In this regard, Ayurveda provides a more personalized treatment method than traditional ED treatment methods. Of particular interest to those that suffer from ED, Ayurveda treatments may involve a change in diet, avoidance of tobacco and alcohol, massages using natural oils that work against ED, and the use of herbal aphrodisiacs.

Changes in Lifestyle

As part of your ayurvedic treatment, your practitioner may suggest several lifestyle changes. He or she may suggest alterations to your diet that include drinking more milk, eating nuts like almonds, or eating ghee (a type of clarified butter). Milk is thought of containing high levels of shukra, and increasing your milk intake will increase the level of shukra in your body. In addition to adding foods to your diet, the practitioner will probably also suggest that you stay away from certain foods as well. For example, he or she may suggest that you stay away from foods that make you gassy like potatoes. He or she may also suggest avoiding spicy or bitter foods. In addition to food choices, the practitioner might suggest the avoidance of alcohol or tobacco.

Other Treatment Options

In addition to lifestyle changes, an ayurvedic practitioner may suggest a massage using herbal oils to help with ED. Some of the oils used are cinnamon oil, cubeb oil, jasmine oil, and Indian ginseng oil. You can massage yourself with these oils, or have your partner massage you. You can also add these oils to a bath to immerse your body in it. Other than massages, breathing exercises and meditation can be included into your ayurvedic treatment.

Vajikarana

An important component within an ayurvedic treatment for ED is the use of herbal medications. This treatment is referred to as *vajikarana*, which literally means "the vigor of a horse." It's basically the use of natural aphrodisiacs, and is intended to strengthen your virility. It helps you feel satisfied and content. The effects of using these herbal treatments include increased libido, ability to achieve erection, relief from stress and anxiety, and increase sexual potency. Ayurvedic herbal treatments usually center on a formulation that mixes several ingredients to create the desired effect. There are many different formulations that vary in potency. The most common formulations are: Vrihani Gutika, Vrishya Gutika, Vajikaranam Ghritam, Upatyakari Shashtikadi Gutika, Medadi Yog, Makardhwaja Gold, and Shatavari Kalpa. The most potent formulation is Vrihani Gutika. The practitioner takes your life signature into consideration when prescribing a particular formulation.

One of the primary herbal remedies used in vajikarana formulations is ashwaghanda, otherwise known as Indian ginseng. The Sanskrit name means "horse smell" because the herb has a horse-like smell. It helps to relieve stress and anxiety, increase blood flow, and increase virility.

Another common herbal ingredient in ayurvedic formulations is bhadra. Bhadra is also known as horny goat weed because goats eat this herb during mating season. It aids in increased blood flow, libido, and testosterone levels. Recent studies have indicated that horny goat weed works in the same manner as prescription ED drugs without adverse side effects.

A final herbal ingredient that is used in formulations is kapikacchu. A common name for this legume is velvet bean. In addition to its aphrodisiac properties, velvet bean aids in reducing blood pressure and cholesterol. It also stimulates the increase of neurotransmitters. Velvet bean has been proven to increase testosterone levels. Also, studies have determined that velvet bean's level of L-Dopa inhibits the effects of prolactin, a hormone in your body that decreases the chances of achieving an erection.

Modern Confirmation of an Ancient Cure

Modern medicine's fascination with Ayurveda only confirms that the ancient healing art has some fundamentals of truth behind it. Recent studies have proven this time and again. But you shouldn't rely on someone else's word on the subject. If you feel that Ayurveda presents you with a vital option for alternative treatment for ED, then speak to your healthcare provider about it.

Chapter 8: Other Alternative Methods for Treating ED

So far you've discussed several alternative treatment methods for treating ED that are safe and natural. While these methods are very inclusive in approach, there are several other things that you can do to complement these methods. By adding these additional steps, you will increase your chance of curing your ED for good. These steps are things that you can do at home to promote and maintain your virility. As with the other treatment methods offered in this book, these additional steps are safe and natural.

Aerobic Exercise
With the issue of blood flow being relevant to ED, participating in regular aerobic exercise can help

you with your ED. Aerobic exercise has been proven to promote stress reduction, increase blood flow, increase oxygen delivery, release endorphins, and increase energy and stamina.

To achieve these benefits of aerobic activity, you need to participate in aerobic activity for at least 30 minutes a day for at least 4 days a week. The more you exercise, the better you will feel. When beginning, it's better to start off with small increments and increase the amount of time as you go. If you want to begin an aerobic exercise routine, you should consult your healthcare provider first. Being safe with aerobic activity is important to your health.

One of the many positive traits of aerobic exercise is that you don't have to buy expensive equipment to participate. As a matter of fact, you don't have to buy any equipment for walking daily for 30 minutes, other than having proper shoes. Walking is a great example of aerobic activity. A regular walking routine will achieve the aerobic benefits that you desire. In addition to walking, you can swim or bicycle. Choose the form of exercise that is best for you. Participate in activities that you enjoy so that you will want to continue the regimen.

Getting the Proper Amount of Rest

Your body can't function properly if it's fatigued. A lack of proper sleep can cause your immune system to malfunction. It can also increase the amount of stress and anxiety you may already be experiencing. Your body rejuvenates itself during the sleep cycle. If your sleep pattern is disrupted, your body cannot heal itself properly.

Due to the causes of your ED, you may not be able to sleep restfully. There are many different natural methods that can help you restore your sleep patterns to a healthy level. If you're having trouble sleeping, you can try deep breathing exercises before going to bed. Or you can meditate. Both of these methods are effective if you can't slow your thoughts down enough to enter into a healthy sleeping pattern. You may also want to consider the condition of your mattress or pillow. Getting comfortable is important for entering into a healthy sleep pattern. Other environmental factors that may disrupt sleep are the amount of ambient light in your bedroom and any noisy distractions within or near your bedroom. Making adjustments to these two factors or using methods to block out these distractions can help you achieve a more restful sleep.

Modifying Your Diet

Your diet can be a cause of your ED. If you eat a diet rich in fat and cholesterol, you could be increasing the chances of your experiencing ED. These types of foods are conducive to high blood pressure and clogged arteries. Obesity has been linked to ED causation as well. By improving your diet, you can improve blood flow.

Studies have shown that ED is uncommon among men who eat a Mediterranean diet. This diet includes fruits, vegetables, nuts, fish, and whole grains. Eating green vegetables is helpful because of the nitrates that these vegetables contain. Nitrates are known to increase blood flow. You can also drink beet juice to achieve the same effect. Dark chocolate is something else that you can eat. The flavonoids in dark chocolate help lower blood pressure and decrease cholesterol. Eating tomatoes and pink grapefruit could help you as well. Both of these fruits contain lycopene, which aids in blood circulation. Finally, oysters have long been thought of to be an aphrodisiac. Recent research indicates that the reasoning behind this belief is the fact that oysters and other shellfish contain high levels of zinc. Zinc has been shown to aid in the production of testosterone.

There are many different things that you can eat that can help increase blood circulation, induce relaxation, and relieve stress and anxiety. The key to modifying your diet is to eat healthy. A healthy diet will benefit you, not only with your ED but in your overall health to boot. Smart eating is always a good choice for your body, whether or not you're experiencing ED. But if you are experiencing ED, a healthy diet will help you overcome it and will help prevent its return.

Taking Supplements
In addition to eating a healthy diet, taking daily supplements may help as well. These supplements are meant to be a healthy alternative to prescription ED drugs. But just because these supplements are alternatives to prescription medications, this doesn't mean that you should take them without knowing about them. Discuss these alternatives with your healthcare provider, so that you are informed as to what options are best for you in light of your medical history and current state of health.

L-arginine
L-arginine is an amino acid that is present in your body. L-arginine has been shown to increase blood flow and lower blood pressure. It does so by creating nitric oxide, a chemical that causes the

blood vessels to open wider. L-arginine is found naturally in red meat, poultry, fish, and dairy products. Pistachios have also been reported to be high in L-arginine. It can also be synthesized and taken as a supplement.

DHEA

Another supplement that you can take for ED is DHEA. DHEA, or dehydroepiandrosterone, is a hormone that is produced by your adrenal glands. It can also be synthesized from wild yam or soy. It is known to be converted by your body into testosterone. One study showed that men with ED were likely to have low levels of DHEA.

Saw Palmetto

A third supplement that has been used for treating erectile dysfunction is saw palmetto. Saw palmetto comes from the fruit of a palm tree. Saw palmetto has been used in the treatment of an enlarged prostate and has been shown to cure ED that is caused by an enlarged prostate. Furthermore, taking saw palmetto has been linked to an increase in sexual drive.

Maca

Finally, maca is a supplement that you may want to try in an effort to rid yourself of ED. Maca is a root found in the Andes that is akin to a turnip but tastes like a potato. This root has been processed into an herbal supplement. Maca has long been considered an aphrodisiac. The benefits of taking maca supplements include increased libido, increased stamina, and reduced anxiety. Maca has been shown to not increase testosterone levels. This lack of hormonal changes makes maca a safe choice because it won't cause you to experience any negative side effects.

Curing, Prevention, and Maintenance

These healthy alternative options for ED aren't only useful in curing ED. No, they go further than this to help prevent ED. Living healthy with proper exercise, diet, and taking healthy supplements provides a backdrop for an increase in vitality. Such lifestyle choices also help to maintain this vitality.

Healthy living is about creating a balance within your choices. It's about choosing activities that support a healthy lifestyle. For your body to function at peak performance, you have to keep your body healthy. Your body functions holistically, so every choice you make in one area affects the whole body. Maintaining a healthy lifestyle can cure ED and prevent future experiences with ED. And you can do this in a manner that is safe and natural by using the methods described above.

.

Chapter 9: Choosing What's Right for You

ED is a common condition amongst men. Even though this statement is true, that doesn't mean that you have to rely on a cure that is common amongst other ED sufferers. In actuality, it's doubtful as to whether or not there is such a thing as a common cure for ED. Sure, there are treatment methods that are relied on more than others, but no single cure works 100% of the time.

Your Body is Unique

The reason that no single cure is 100% effective for curing ED is because your body is unique. Even though the general makeup of your body is the same as every other male body, the specifics of your body are unique to you. For example, your medical history is unique. Your chemical makeup is also different. Your psychological/emotional condition is unique. There are so many specific traits that combine to make you who you are as an individual.

An Effective Treatment Plan is Tailored for Your Body

That's the mystery of the human body. We are in so many ways similar, yet in so many ways different. What works as a treatment method for others may not work for you. Any effective treatment plan will take into consideration the specifics of your current life situation and the specifics of your body makeup.

You will also want an ED treatment plan that is holistic in its approach. ED isn't just about the body. It affects your whole being. Your ED treatment plan should take into consideration how your ED is affecting your whole person and address all of these issues.

While traditional ED treatment plans often take your physical and psychological state into consideration, they may not address your spirit. Your ED plan needs to take into consideration your beliefs and values. If you find that traditional treatment plans are incongruent with your beliefs and values, you should consider alternative ED treatment methods.

Improving Your Quality of Life

Alternative ED treatment methods take into consideration your mind, body, and spirit. The goal of alternative treatment methods is to not only treat your ED, but to improve your overall quality of life. ED affects more than just your sexual experience. ED affects your relationships, your ability to focus in your daily life, and your ability to make sound choices. ED causes a drain in your life energy. Alternative ED treatments take your life energy into consideration.

A Healthcare Provider Who Understands Your Wants

How you treat your ED is your choice. You don't have to choose a treatment because it's right for someone else. You need to choose an ED treatment because it's right for *you*. Yes, you should consult your healthcare provider concerning options for treating your ED. You should be honest during this communication and express your desires for ED treatment options. If your healthcare professional is not an advocate of alternative ED treatments, feel free to find a healthcare provider that supports your beliefs. Alternative medicine is being embraced more and more today and finding a healthcare professional who values alternative medicine in the same way that you do shouldn't be difficult.

Take Control of Your ED Treatment and Take Control of Your Life

It may take some effort to find a healthcare professional who promotes alternative medicine, but honoring your choices is worth the effort. Staying committed to your choice in alternative medicine is taking control of your ED treatment. Taking control of your ED treatment allows you to take back control of your life. Ultimately, that's the heart of alternative medicine: you being in touch with your body and bringing balance to your mind, body, and spirit. You don't have to be limited by your ED. You can be freed from ED through alternative medicine treatments. This freedom will allow you to increase your confidence, focus, and stamina while removing physical and psychological blocks that stand in the way of your contentment. Your life contains so much more than just your sexual performance. Alternative medicine ED treatments allow you to embrace the full life that you are meant to live in a manner that is safe and natural. Choose alternative ED treatments and choose to honor your life.

Conclusion

Thank you again for purchasing this book!
I hope this book was able to help you to achieve
the quality of life that you desire through natural
and safe treatments for your ED with alternative
methods.

Remember, your body is unique and so is your
experience. Your ED treatment plan should take
that uniqueness into consideration. If you truly
want an ED treatment plan that takes your quality
of life into consideration, speak to your healthcare
provider regarding alternative treatment methods.

The next step is to enjoy the fullness of life that is
yours to enjoy now that you're free from ED. Take
control of your life by determining your ED

treatment plan. You don't have to suffer from ED. You don't even have to suffer through a treatment plan that you're not comfortable with. It's your body. Return it to the proper balance and enjoy all of your experiences again in a manner that is wholesome and natural.

Finally, if you enjoyed this book, then I'd like to ask you for a favor. Would you be kind enough to leave a review for this book on Amazon? It'd be greatly appreciated!

Thank you and good luck!

Other books by Michael Cesar:

Tantric Love —The Sacred Union Of Souls

Improve Your Love Life And Your Relationship with Tantra—By Michael Cesar

The union of two people on more than a physical level is the ultimate goal as you read through this book. Once you allow yourself to be one with your partner and the divine, you will experience true sexual freedom and lose your inhibitions with your partner.

Success Habits

Kaizen — Improve Your Life and Become Successful by Taking One Small Step at a Time — By Michael Cesar

This book is a dynamic resource for men and women alike to set small, attainable goals that are measurable and maintain a pattern of positive behavior. "Kaizen" means "change for better," and is created to increase your productivity at work as well as at home.

Effortless Manifestation Magic And Miracles

Discover The Single Most Powerful Method Of Manifesting Your Dream Life From Oneness - By Michael Cesar

Within the universe lays a wealth of information that the human mind has only just begun to tap into. Manifesting is one of those sources which are readily available to anyone who seeks to obtain the miracles that the universe is waiting to impart on every individual. Similar to prayer and meditation, manifesting is a personal journey into the magic of self-discovery and a unique oneness with the world around us.

Ayurveda Weight Loss

The Ultimate Guide to Successful Ayurvedic Detox and Weight Loss — By Michael Cesar

This book covers the cleansing/detoxification process, the Ayurvedic diet, the lifestyle changes, as well as tips and aids for daily life and maintaining commitment to your weight loss goals and personal goals.

The Natural Cure for Erectile Dysfunction

How to Cure Erectile Dysfunction And Impotency Permanently In The Comfort of your own Home By Following These Simple And Easy Proven Methods—By Michael Cesar

Discover how to finally overcome Erectile Dysfunction, impotency, premature ejaculation, inhibited ejaculation, sexual inexperience, pornography addictions, or sexual addiction as well as other sexual issues.

CPSIA information can be obtained
at www.ICGtesting.com
Printed in the USA
LVOW04s1150191116
513697LV00010B/503/P